GIVING AND RECEIVING CRITICISM

Your Key to Interpersonal Success

Patti Hathaway

A FIFTY-MINUTE™ SERIES BOOK

CRISP PUBLICATIONS, INC.
Menlo Park, California

GIVING AND RECEIVING CRITICISM
Your Key to Interpersonal Success

Patti Hathaway

CREDITS
Editor: **Anne Knight**
Design/Typesetting: **Interface Studio**
Cover Design: **Carol Harris**
Artwork: **Ralph Mapson**

English language Crisp books are distributed worldwide. Our major international distributors include:

CANADA: Reid Publishing Ltd., Box 69559—109 Thomas St., Oakville, Ontario Canada L6J 7R4. TEL: (416) 842-4428, FAX: (416) 842-9327

AUSTRALIA: Career Builders, P. O. Box 1051, Springwood, Brisbane, Queensland, Australia 4127. TEL: 841-1061, FAX: 841-1580

NEW ZEALAND: Career Builders, P. O. Box 571, Manurewa, Auckland, New Zealand. TEL: 266-5276, FAX: 266-4152

JAPAN: Phoenix Associates Co., Mizuho Bldg. 2-12-2, Kami Osaki, Shinagawa-Ku, Tokyo 141, Japan. TEL: 3-443-7231, FAX: 3-443-7640

Selected Crisp titles are also available in other languages. Contact International Rights Manager Tim Polk at (800) 442-7477 for more information.

Library of Congress Catalog Card Number 89-82345
Hathaway, Patti
Giving and Receiving Criticism
ISBN 1-56052-023-X

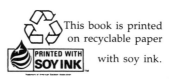

This book is printed on recyclable paper with soy ink.

PRINTED WITH
SOY INK

TO THE READER

Have you ever felt like screaming because you were criticized unfairly, yet you weren't quite sure how to respond, so you just kept quiet? Or you really wanted to give someone negative criticism but you weren't sure how to phrase it so he or she wouldn't take it personally?

All of us, at one time or another, have been in uncomfortable situations because of criticism. This book is designed to help you assess your strengths and weaknesses in both giving and taking criticism.

Handling criticism is an essential skill for any professional. Given properly, criticism can turn a non-productive employee around. Taken well, it increases our chances for growth and development.

There are no two ways about it: Criticism is here to stay. It's just a matter of how we cope with it. This is a book for someone who wants to reap the benefits of learning how to give and take criticism more effectively. Come join us as we learn some practical techniques for increasing our interpersonal effectiveness!

Best Wishes for Success!

Patti Hathaway

Patti Hathaway

> "A soft answer turns away wrath, but harsh words cause quarrels."
> Proverbs 15:1

ABOUT THE AUTHOR

Patti Hathaway is a results-oriented speaker, trainer, and corporate consultant. She brings a fresh, dynamic approach based on the business savvy and insights gained from working with different organizations including manufacturing, insurance, government, high technology, research, education, health care, agriculture, as well as civic, community, and church groups.

Patti delivers more than 120 seminars annually across the United States on such topics as communication skills, handling with difficult people, and leadership development. She is also a speaker with Fred Pryor Seminars. Selected as the State of Ohio's 1988 ''Outstanding Young Career Woman'' by the Business and Professional Women's Association (BPW), Patti received her Bachelor of Arts degree from Calvin College in Grand Rapids, Michigan and her Masters degree in Education and Training from the Ohio State University.

Patti is an active member of the National Speakers Association and has served on the board of directors of the Ohio Speakers Forum, Central Ohio American Society of Training & Development, Capitol City BPW, and Calvin College Alumni Association. She is listed in the *1986-87 Outstanding Young Women in America* and the *1989 Who's Who in American Christian Leadership* directories.

Patti welcomes your comments and questions. You can reach her at The Hathaway Group, 1016 Woodglen Road, Westerville, Ohio 43081-3236, (614) 523-3633.

ACKNOWLEDGEMENTS

Special thanks to my dear friend Debra Aungst and to my colleague Barbara Braham for helping critique and edit the draft of this book.

Thanks also to my husband Jim, for being both my best critic and favorite fan through the years.

CONTENTS

PART I
HOW TO TAKE CRITICISM

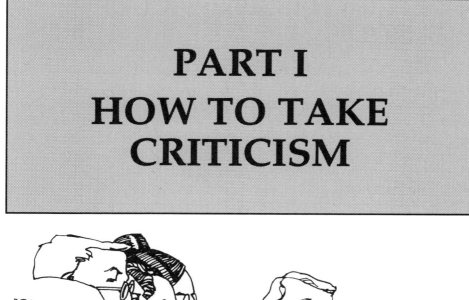

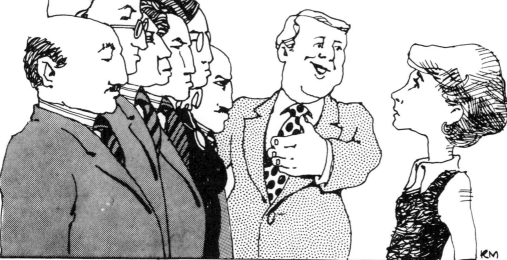

*"YOUR COLLEAGUES WOULD LIKE TO SHARE THEIR
REACTIONS TO YOUR PROJECT, MS. JONES!"*

The only way to avoid criticism is to do nothing, say nothing, be nothing.

Elbert Hubbard

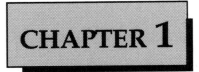

WHY IS CRITICISM DIFFICULT TO HANDLE?

When it comes to criticism, most of us believe it is more blessed to give than to receive. Yet, valid criticism from others, when properly given, can make the difference between success and failure in our lives. It provides us with feedback on what's working and what's not. Why, then, do we find criticism so difficult to handle? Perhaps it is because most of us define criticism as Webster does in the dictionary, ''the act of criticizing unfavorably.'' We often view criticism as something totally negative. Criticism is defined as ''the art of evaluating or analyzing with knowledge and propriety...'' Unfortunately, many of the people in our lives who criticize us do so without full knowledge and it is often delivered in an improper manner.

Criticism is an indispensable part of our lives. If we can understand and use it, criticism can empower us to become better people. Why, then, do so many of us resist taking full advantage of what can be such an enormous benefit?

One of the reasons why we tend to resist criticism is that a good part of our self-image is based on how others view us. When we find out that someone sees us in a less than positive light, we can feel devastated.

The world over, people tend to like to hear what is consistent with their own views and to resist ideas contrary to their belief structures. If we knew we were doing something ineffectively, wouldn't we automatically try to improve the deficiency? Criticism implies that we could be wrong. What could be more personal and threatening? It takes an open mind to be able to listen to an opposing view.

PARENT MESSAGES AND CRITICISM

Our past affects how we handle criticism. Much of our past is buried in the messages we received as youngsters. Some people internalize their parents' expectations and beliefs about themselves, doing everything in their power to gain approval from their parents and later from others. Often they come to criticize themselves far more harshly than their parents ever did.

Following is an exercise designed by Madelyn Burley-Allen, author of *Managing Assertively* (Wiley Press, 1983). It will help you analyze childhood messages you may have encountered and their ramifications to you as an adult.

Exercise: Parent Messages

1. Check any messages that you received as a child.

☐ "Don't be angry."

☐ "Be perfect."

☐ "Children should be seen and not heard."

☐ "What will other people think?"

☐ "Don't make trouble."

☐ "If you can't say anything nice, don't say anything."

☐ "Don't interrupt."

☐ "Grit your teeth and bear it."

☐ "Always finish what you start."

☐ "Don't fight back."

☐ "Older people know better than you."

☐ "Be careful or you might get hurt."

PARENT MESSAGE EXERCISE (Continued)

2. List any other messages you received as a child:

_____

_____

_____

3. Pick three of the messages you received as a child and analyze how they affect your behavior as an adult and how you respond to criticism:

MESSAGE   RAMIFICATIONS

_____

_____

_____

_____

_____

TWO "PARENT" MESSAGES

Typically, when we leave home parents do not take us aside and tell us that it's time for us to choose which values to keep and which to discard. When something does go wrong, we replay our "parent tapes"—the messages we received as kids—pointing out that our parents were right all along. Let's look at two parental messages and how they might affect our ability to handle criticism as adults.

PARENT MESSAGE #1

One message very familiar to many adults is; "What will other people think?" This message is especially prevalent among people who grew up in small towns or who had parents in prominent positions (i.e. minister/rabbi, doctor, mayor, principal, etc.).

Some of the ramifications of this message might be:

1. A need as adults for others to approve of our behavior; therefore, any criticism of our behavior is taken personally.

2. A lack of risk-taking behavior for fear others may not approve of our action. If we make no decisions in life, we will make no mistakes and, therefore, can guard ourselves against criticism.

3. Similarly, an adult with this childhood message will probably take a reactive stance in life, always waiting for others to act first.

As an adult affected by that message, you may have learned to do everything in your power to get others to accept and approve of you. You may, in fact, have fallen into what some call an "approval trap." The harder we try to please people, the more unhappy we become when we sense that others are still dissatisfied. What is more rational is to recognize that we will never please everyone. We must begin walking to the beat of our own drum.

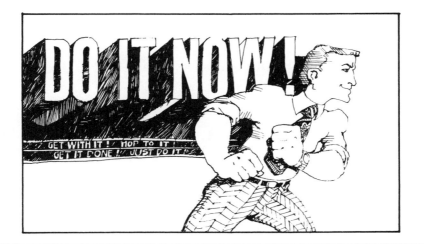

What we are may be our parents' fault; what we remain is our responsibility.

Anonymous

PARENT MESSAGE #2

Another message familiar from childhood is; ''If you can't say anything nice, don't say anything.'' The ramifications of this message may include:

1. Not giving criticism, because what you have to say may not be perceived as ''nice'' by the recipient.

2. The belief that other people do not have the right to criticize you but only provide feedback that is ''nice'' or positive.

3. The belief that criticism that is not ''nice'' or positive is ''bad'' and that nothing good can possibly result from negative feedback.

4. The belief that it is better to hold back expressing (repress) negative feelings than to share them; therefore, you withhold criticism of others.

It may be particularly difficult to take criticism as an adult if you received a lot of it as a child. As kids, we were vulnerable, because we could neither resist criticism nor defend ourselves.

What we should realize is that criticism has *two* interactors—one giver and one receiver. It is not just something we must ''take,'' but something we can respond to and interact with.

A CHILD LIVES WHAT HE LEARNS

If a child lives with criticism, He learns to condemn.

If a child lives with ridicule, He learns to be shy.

If a child lives with hostility, He learns to fight.

If a child lives with shame, He learns to feel guilty.

If a child lives with tolerance, He learns to be patient.

If a child lives with encouragement, He learns confidence.

If a child lives with praise, He learns appreciation.

If a child lives with fairness, He learns justice.

If a child lives with security, He learns to have faith.

If a child lives with approval, He learns to like himself.

If a child lives with acceptance and friendship, He learns to find love in the world.

Author Unknown

GENDER, SELF-IMAGE, AND CRITICISM

Research indicates that our ability to handle criticism is often related to our level of self-confidence. Men and women between the ages of 18-34 are more highly sensitive to criticism, because they are still in the process of developing a sense of identity.

The expression "women take things too personally" also tends to be true. In part, because many men grew up playing team sports, they are accustomed to receiving feedback on their performance and view it as a way to find out how to meet performance standards. Women, on the other hand, often grew up with the mistaken view that criticism meant something must be wrong with them. All of us need to recognize that criticism and disapproval are *not* synonymous.

An interesting research study was conducted by several psychologists who wanted to examine differences between men and women and how the two sexes internalize positive and negative feedback and experiences. Specifically, they explored how men and women view success and failure.

The participants were divided into same-sex groups—the men worked together and the women worked together. Both groups were assigned the same task. The first task was to assemble a puzzle that was impossible to put together—it was rigged and both groups were doomed to "failure."

When the researchers asked the men why they couldn't complete the puzzle, what would you guess the men said? The men replied that there was something wrong *with the puzzle*, that it was "rigged" and "impossible to complete."

The same scenario was repeated with the group of women. After the women struggled with the puzzle for some time, the researchers asked them why they couldn't complete the puzzle. How do you think the women responded? They weren't sure why they couldn't complete the puzzle . . . maybe if they'd had more time? perhaps they weren't smart enough? and puzzles really weren't their forte? It was striking that the women simply assumed that fault lay with them and not with the puzzle!

GENDER, SELF-IMAGE, AND CRITICISM (Continued)

The interesting difference between these men and women and their response to negative feedback is that the men tended to externalize failure and the women tended to internalize failure. Think about practical, everyday examples with criticism. If a man doesn't do well in a game of golf or softball or any sport, for that matter, what does he tend to do? Often he will blame the golf clubs, the officials, the playing field, etc. Often, men have difficulty admitting that perhaps they are not quite the athletes they once were.

In contrast, women tend to internalize criticism immediately. Obviously they are not any good at puzzles, or at writing reports, or whatever. Often, they will not even question the source or the possibility that the criticism is unfounded.

The second part of the study was equally interesting. This time, the researchers looked at how men and women attribute their success. Both groups were given a very simple puzzle and both quickly assembled it.

When asked to what they attributed their success, the men replied that completing puzzles was one of their talents. They internalized their success and took credit for it. The women, on the other hand, replied that they were ''just lucky'' or that the puzzle was ''easy.'' They externalized their success, crediting the simple puzzle, not their own puzzle-solving ability.

The Simmons Market Research Bureau, in coordination with Bright Enterprises, conducted a study of attitudes towards criticism of 11,000 adults throughout the United States. Their study confirms the results above. Although 71% of the men surveyed indicated that they were ''hard'' or ''extremely hard'' on themselves, 85% of the women claimed high levels of self-criticism.

Regardless of gender, we need to begin looking at how we set our performance standards and make sure we are being realistic. Both men and women need to listen to praise as well as to negative criticism, to use an objective measure to see how they are meeting standards, and, if indicated, to uncover what they're doing wrong. To internalize or externalize negative feedback or criticism automatically is to deprive ourselves of the objectivity we need to evaluate criticism and its source realistically. When we accurately attribute our performance to our abilities, we build a base of information about ourselves that will help us set and meet our future expectations.

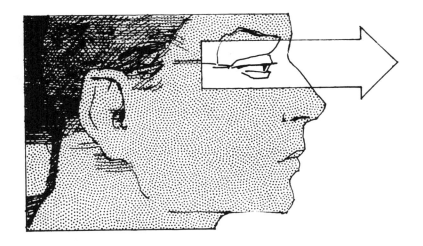

If I am not for myself, who will be for me?
If I am not for others, who am I for?
And if not now, when?

The Talmud

EXERCISE: SELF-IMAGE INDEX

Let's take a look at our self-image and discover how vulnerable we are to our own criticism.

Self-Image Index

1. Rate yourself on how well the following statements apply to you, using the following scale: (1) Usually applies, (2) Sometimes applies, (3) Rarely applies, (4) Never applies.

    _____ It is not easy for me to tell my friends that I am good at something.

    _____ I feel hurt and humiliated when someone makes a joke at my expense.

    _____ I am not accepted by most people I meet.

    _____ I don't want to cause trouble for others, so I'd rather do something myself than ask for help.

    _____ I have trouble saying no to requests made of me.

    _____ I fear others say bad things behind my back.

    _____ If I tell others what I really feel, they may get angry.

    _____ I don't want to get involved or I might get hurt.

    _____ I do not have much self-confidence when it comes to new and unfamiliar situations.

    _____ I avoid situations where there might be conflict.

    _____ When things happen outside of my control, I usually take the blame.

    _____ I don't want to make waves.

    _____ TOTAL SCORE

The lower your score, the more self-doubts and self-criticism you probably experience. In all likelihood, you are your own worst critic. You need to begin examining the performance standards you measure yourself against realistically. The skills to handle these problems are outlined in Chapters Two and Six.

A lot of our ability to handle criticism is based on our self-image and the guilt we experience from childhood messages. Yet, how can we counteract those two aspects, so ingrained in our very being?

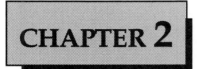

COUNTERACTING SELF-CRITICISM WITH POSITIVE SELF-TALK

One powerful way to counteract self-critical messages is to change how we think and what we believe about ourselves and our situation. Our beliefs have tremendous impact on the outcome of any situation. Eleanor Roosevelt said memorably and truly, that ''No one can make you feel inferior without your consent.'' It all comes back to our beliefs. If we can change our beliefs, often we can change how we perceive criticism. A simple formula to demonstrate this is:

$$A + B = C, \text{ where}$$

A = Activating Event

B = Belief about that event

C = Consequence/outcome

Two people can encounter the same activating event of a traffic jam and have two completely opposite outcomes. Becky is a ''Type A'' driver who races to each traffic light and is always speeding. When she encounters a traffic snarl, she blames the traffic jam on all the ''incompetent'' drivers out there. As a result, she weaves in and out of traffic and takes side roads to try and bypass the jam. The consequence for Becky is that by the time she reaches her office at 8:06 a.m. she is experiencing high blood pressure and fatigue.

George, in contrast to Becky, always drives at the speed limit and considers himself a good driver. When he encounters a traffic snarl, he believes that it is simply a matter of time before it is cleared and enjoys the extra time provided him with an opportunity to listen to his favorite radio station. The consequence? George arrives at the office at 8:09 a.m. relaxed and ready to begin the day's work.

The important thing to note in this example is that the activating event was identical, yet the outcome was completely different. The reason? Becky and George had very different beliefs about traffic.

BELIEFS ABOUT CRITICISM

Let's look at your beliefs about criticism. If you believe that all criticism is negative and means that you are a failure, then the outcome for you of being criticized will be a rejection of yourself and your ability, which may result in an inability to move forward, change, grow, and develop. In fact, you may stagnate, never breaking down the walls with which you have protectively surrounded yourself.

If, on the other hand, you accept and welcome criticism as a vehicle for learning, then the outcome of criticism will be much less stressful, for you are free to accept or reject it.

An irony of criticism is that the more you resist it, the more it becomes a problem. The more accepting you are towards criticism and its inevitability, the better you can use criticism to your advantage.

Another way to explain the impact of our beliefs is to examine our ''self-talk.'' Self-talk is the stream-of-conscious thoughts (beliefs) that reflect our attitude towards events in our lives. Self-talk and our beliefs often make for self-fulfilling prophecy. Therefore, it is vital that we control what we say to ourselves.

Negative self-talk can contribute to our feeling overwhelmed and defeated by those who criticize us. If we allow someone else to determine how we feel about ourselves, we give him or her the power to control our reaction to criticism. We must realize that criticism is neither in itself negative nor positive unless we attribute meaning to it. We *do* possess complete control over the meaning we attribute to criticism and, therefore, how we will respond to it.

> If you don't change your beliefs, your life will be like this forever. Is that good news?
>
> Robert Anthony

EXERCISE: SELF-TALK ATTITUDES

Self-talk begins inside each one of us. We cannot control others criticizing us.
However, we *can* control what we say to ourselves while being criticized
by others.

1. Some of the attitudes that contribute to negative self-talk are provided below.
   Check the statements that are true for you:

   ☐   Since I do not receive perfect ratings in every area of my latest
   performance appraisal, I see myself as a failure in my job.

   ☐   I attribute successes to something other than my own abilities or talent.

   ☐   My child received a ''C'' in math on his or her last report card and I
   blame myself for not having spent enough time with him/her.

   ☐   A co-worker has been acting a bit funny lately and I assume it was
   something I said or did.

   ☐   The presentation I gave at the department staff meeting last month did
   not come off as well as I would have liked, so I am convinced that my
   next presentation will also be a failure.

   ☐   I find myself labeling myself instead of describing a mistake I have
   made...i.e. ''I'm such a jerk!'' ''How could I have been such a fool?!''
   ''Only an idiot would have...''

   ☐   My boss corrects an error in the proposal I just submitted, and I find
   myself feeling incompetent in proposal writing as a result of the
   criticism.

2. Write down one or two negative self-talk statements you make to yourself
   when under pressure or when you have just been criticized.

   _____

   _____

   _____

3. Analyze the statements you just wrote down rationally and rewrite them to be
   positive and proactive. Begin each statement with ''I am...''

   _____

   _____

   _____

POSITIVE SELF-TALK EXAMPLES

Below are two of the self-talk examples rewritten to be more positive:

> "I am good at what I do as a _____. In my recent performance evaluation, I received almost all "4's" and "5's," so I plan to continue my current levels of performance in those areas. In area _____, I received a "3," which is "average or meets standards." This is how I plan to bring my rating up to at least a "4" next evaluation..."
>
> "I am well prepared for my presentation at this week's department meeting and know that it will be a success."
>
> Please note that in these two examples, the first one is said to oneself after the fact and the second example is to be repeated to yourself before a stressful event.

We must realize that we can be very "SNIOP" (Susceptible to the Negative Influences of Other People). Yet we all have control over our beliefs and thoughts. No one can make us feel angry, inferior, frustrated, put-down, unless we allow ourselves to feel that way. It is a good thing for each of us to examine whether or not we want to *become* what we say to ourselves. We often hear the comment "you are what you eat," but far more important is "you are what you think."

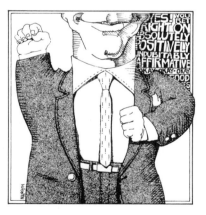

> Our THOUGHTS become ACTIONS, which develop HABITS, eventually building our CHARACTER.
>
> Author unknown

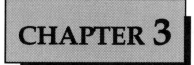

CHAPTER 3

HOW DO I HANDLE CRITICISM?

The Simmons/Bright study on criticism found that we resent receiving criticism most from our in-laws (24%), mate (22%), and subordinates (21%). We handle it best from teachers, friends, father, or boss.

Interestingly, we consider it most important to take corrective action when criticized by our boss (72%) and mate (62%) and least important to take corrective action when criticized by our in-laws and siblings. Corresponding with those results, we will actually try to change our behavior when criticized by our boss (61%) and mate (54%).

We are hurt most by criticism that questions our integrity (85%) and our job performance (74%). Women were found to react more sensitively than men in all the situations described.

Often, the difficulty we face in handling criticism lies in the fact that the criticism is at least partially true. If the criticism were absurd, it wouldn't trouble us. However, even if the criticism is poorly given, it forces us to examine our behavior and draw some conclusions.

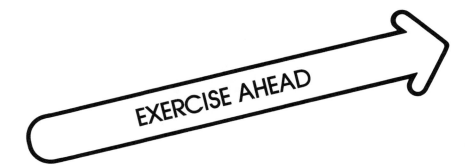

EXERCISE AHEAD

EXERCISE: SELF-ASSESSMENT IN HANDLING CRITICISM

1. Place a "plus" (+) by those situations you handle appropriately, a "minus" (−) by those you avoid handling, and a "zero" (0) by those you handle but not well.

   _____ In a department meeting, you make an important statement that everyone ignores.

   _____ Your boss criticizes your job performance.

   _____ Your spouse criticizes your appearance.

   _____ You hear from a colleague that your boss is upset about a comment you made in yesterday's staff meeting.

   _____ Someone criticizes you for something you know you didn't do.

   _____ A colleague makes an off-handed negative comment about a project of which you are in charge.

   _____ Things haven't been going well for you lately, you are feeling "down," and your office mate criticizes you for your "bad attitude."

   _____ A manager from another department sends you a memo outlining his/her criticism of your latest idea.

   _____ You are criticized in a gender-related manner, i.e., "That's just like a female."

   _____ You complete an assignment to the best of your ability and are told you could have done a better job.

   _____ You apply for a new job and are turned down.

   _____ A customer on the phone starts yelling at you for something for which you are not responsible.

2. Examine those situations that you marked with a "plus" (+) and list the actions you took in those situations that caused you to be effective:

   _____

   _____

   _____

   _____

   _____

3. Analyze those situations that you marked with a ''minus'' (−) and ''zero'' (0) and write down why those situations are difficult for you to handle and the actions you typically take:

       A. WHY DIFFICULT?   B. TYPICAL RESPONSE

_____

_____

_____

_____

4. Are any of the reasons you listed above in 3A related to your self-image or your parent messages outlined in Chapter 1? If so, what are some patterns you are beginning to notice?

_____

_____

_____

_____

5. What positive self-talk statements can you use to counter your negative beliefs and messages?

_____

_____

_____

_____

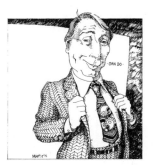

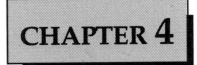

CHAPTER 4

TYPES OF CRITICISM

There are basically three types of criticism that we experience: (1) Valid, or bona fide, criticism, (2) Unjustified, or invalid, criticism, and (3) Criticism that is vague or is simply a difference of opinion.

1. *VALID CRITICISM* is in some ways the most difficult type of criticism for us to handle, because at some point we have to admit it is just. However, one tendency in responding to valid criticism is to give it more heed than necessary, to make it more important than it really is. We must recognize that we all make mistakes. We need to accept ourselves even when we do make mistakes. It is helpful to keep in mind that the more active and fruitful our lives, the more likely we will be to make some mistakes and hence, to receive criticism. Avoiding action simply to avoid the risk of making mistakes is a cowardly and unproductive alternative.

2. *UNJUSTIFIED CRITICISM,* or invalid criticism, may come as a result of our not living up to someone else's fantasy. Often, people do not communicate their expectations of us, and thus, we are vulnerable to disappointing them. But this is their fault, not ours. Moreover, for criticism to be genuinely helpful, it must be expressed in specific, concrete terms, so that we can understand the expectations and take appropriate action if we so choose.

JUST DO IT!

Dr. Hendrie Weisinger, author of *Nobody's Perfect* (Statford Press, 1981) suggests asking yourself several questions to determine whether criticism is valid or invalid:

1. Do I hear the same criticism from more than one person?

2. Does the critic know a great deal about the subject?

3. Are the critic's standards known and reasonable?

4. Is the criticism really about me? (or is the critic merely having a bad day or upset about something else, etc.)

5. How important is it for me to respond to the criticism?

If you respond positively to one or more of the first four questions, the criticism may be valid. If you responded negatively to most of the questions, the criticism is likely to be invalid.

3. The third type of criticism is *VAGUE CRITICISM* or criticism that may simply indicate a difference of opinion. In this type of criticism, the critic is often someone who thinks his/her values and methods of doing something are better than yours. Criticism of this kind may act as an effective cover for more deeply held feelings such as jealousy, fear of the unknown, insecurity, or arrogance. But it is important for us to address this type of criticism as well as the other types, because our critic may have legitimate feelings that need to be worked out. In short, this sort of criticism may suggest more about our critic than it does about us.

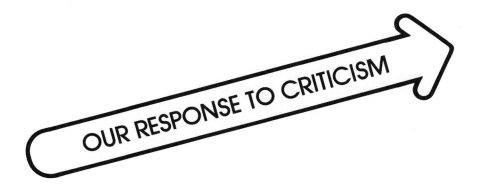

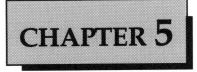

OUR RESPONSE TO CRITICISM

One thing that is good to realize is that, as the recipient of criticism, we have more control than the critic, once the criticism has been delivered. It is then up to us to decide whether we believe the criticism has merit and is worth acting upon.

There are basically three stages we experience when coping with criticism:

STAGE ONE: Awareness Stage

STAGE TWO: Assessment Stage

STAGE THREE: Action Stage

STAGE ONE—AWARENESS

In the AWARENESS stage, we take notice that we are being criticized and our natural instincts take over. We may respond by counterattacking and becoming defensive OR we may become a silent victim and automatically accept the criticism at face value.

Let's look at the pros and cons of these two instinctive responses to criticism.

When we counterattack our critic, we often do so with sarcasm, put downs, or digs. In fact, sometimes, our one-liners are real "zingers," and if we have an audience we may get a big laugh out of them.

Comedians and cartoonists use sarcasm a lot because they can be very funny. As an example, "My wife started to diet when she went from a size nine to a size tent."

The downside of counterattacking is the simple fact that you have not helped to build a relationship but in fact, have resorted to putting your critic down. This does not promote a climate in which you can comfortably continue to talk with your critic, nor your critic with you.

When we counterattack an aggressive critic, we may think we are not affecting that person. However, our critic may not be as thick-skinned as we might have imagined. Often, critical people are as insecure as people who behave passively.

The silent victim or passive approach is no more helpful. If you say nothing or accept the criticism as valid before assessing it, you will appear to have little self-confidence and may lose the respect of others and yourself! Secondly, you may not truly understand what the critic intended by the criticism unless you take time to assess the criticism.

A far better approach to handling with criticism is to be aware that criticism is ''just criticism'' and then move quickly to assessing its merit.

> A man who trims himself to suit everybody will soon whittle himself away.
>
> Charles M. Schwab

STAGE TWO—ASSESS

In Stage 2, you ASSESS how the criticism was delivered, the intention of the critic, and how valid you believe the criticism to be. It is at this point that you may want to ask yourself the five questions outlined earlier to determine whether or not the criticism is valid. Watch, also, for the nonverbal behavior of your critic. You may be able to determine the intensity of his or her feelings and how open he or she will be to the action you decide to take.

> Insults are like bad coins; we cannot help their being offered to us, but we need not take them.
>
> Charles H. Spurgeon

STAGE THREE—ACTION

In the final stage, you decide what ACTION, if any, you want to take with the criticism. Let's examine some ACTION strategies for dealing assertively with criticism.

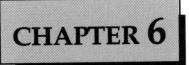

CHAPTER 6

ASSERTIVE TECHNIQUES TO CRITICISM

If we can be assertive while being criticized, it will allow us to remain confident and cool. An assertive approach permits a "win-win" attitude in which you allow your critic to have an opinion while maintaining your own. Manuel J. Smith, author of *When I Say No, I Feel Guilty*, introduced three assertive techniques that have proved invaluable in helping assess and evaluate what action you can take when being criticized.

They are:

Technique #1 FOGGING
Technique #2 ADMITTING THE TRUTH (Negative Assertion)
Technique #3 ASKING FOR FEEDBACK (Negative Inquiry)

We will review each of these techniques by examining the situations and types of criticism in which they are most effective.

Assertively Responding to Unjustified Criticism

The first thing we must do when someone criticizes us invalidly or unjustifiably is to set up a psychological barrier that protects us from taking the criticism personally. One of the foundations mentioned earlier for handling criticism effectively is self-confidence and high self-esteem.

If we believe in ourselves, in our abilities, skills, and knowledge, criticism is much less threatening, and we are able to take it less personally. We must choose to let the criticism have no devastating impact.

TECHNIQUE #1—FOGGING

When faced with unjustified criticism, force yourself to avoid counter criticism or counter manipulating your critic. Instead, use the assertiveness skill, FOGGING.

FOGGING

WHAT IT IS: Calm acknowledgement of the possibility that there may be *some* truth in the criticism.

WHAT IT DOES: Allows you to receive criticism without becoming anxious or defensive. Allows you to be the final judge of what to do about it. You become a ''listener'' instead of a ''reader'' of minds.

RESULT: Like a fog bank, you are unaffected by manipulative, unjustified criticism. After awhile, your critic finds it's no fun to throw things at you.

RESPONSES: ''You could be right about that...''
''You might be right about...''
''What you say makes sense...''
''Perhaps I could...''

Often, unjustified criticism is expressed in broad, general terms, which are unrealistic and untrue and often spoken out of anger. When encountering unjustified criticism, watch out for words like ''always,'' ''never,'' ''all the time,'' and ''every time.''

Let's look at some examples and potential responses:

UNJUSTIFIED CRITICISM	FOGGING RESPONSE
''You're always late.''	''Perhaps I am a bit late this time.''
''Every time you are told about an error, you get defensive.''	''You might be right about my tendency to get defensive. I don't like it when I make errors.''

An easy mistake for people to make with the fogging technique is to ''Yes, but...'' That is, to make a good fogging statement and then add on the reasons why they did what they did. Take the above example, ''Yes, I am late, *but* I've been working on the report you assigned me two days after the deadline...'' A good fogging statement uses active listening skills to paraphrase the criticism while adding a fogging statement.

FOGGING EXAMPLE

Following is a true example of how a shipping/receiving worker in a manufacturing plant used the fogging strategy with his fellow workers.

JOE'S CASE

Joe was incessantly teased about the size of his nose and how it got in the way of his work. Joe's typical response was to get physically violent when teased. He would run the hi-low machine into the wooden storage crates and punch boxes with his fists. His co-workers loved the rise they got out of Joe by teasing him about something beyond his control. How many of us have control over the size of our nose?

Joe decided he would employ the fogging technique when teased about the size of his nose. This is how he replied to his fellow workers' jibes:

TEASING COMMENT	JOE'S FOGGING REPLY
"Joe, would you mind moving out of the way, we can't see the load 'cuz' your nose is in the way."	"Perhaps my nose is blocking your view, let me move for you."

After about a week of fogging, Joe reported to the assertiveness class that his co-workers said to him, "What are you learning in that class? You're not much fun anymore." One result of fogging is that his critics found him less fun to criticize!

One of the greatest benefits to fogging is that it forces you to *listen* to your critic instead of automatically reacting to his/her comments. Secondly, after you have handled the situation, you can decide whether or not the criticism has any merit and whether or not to take any action. In Joe's case, he decided that fogging was a lot less expensive and painful than nose surgery!

If you choose not to use the fogging technique, then you have several other options: (1) Grin and bear it, (2) Ignore it (but watch out for your nonverbal reactions, which may give away your true feelings, and (3) Disagree politely. Always keep in mind that when handling with unjustified criticism, you need to consider the critic. To what degree is the criticism a reflection of your critic's personality and motivation?

EXERCISE: FOGGING

1. Write down potential fogging responses to the following situations:

   A. Your boss comes in and says, ''Why are you always late to our staff meetings? I expected more from you and hoped that you would set an example for the rest of the group.''

   _____

   _____

   B. A co-worker complains to you that you always seem to get what you want from the boss. ''What's the deal?'' he asks.

   _____

   _____

   C. One of the tackiest dressers at work looks at your new suit and sarcastically remarks that it looks like you bought it at the local thrift shop.

   _____

   _____

2. Write down two situations in which you have been criticized unjustifiably. Think through some potential fogging responses to those criticisms.

   INVALID CRITICISM   FOGGING RESPONSE

   (1) _____   _____

   _____   _____

   (2) _____   _____

   _____   _____

Potential Responses to Sitatutions A-C:

A: ''What you say makes sense. I probably should be on time to staff meetings if I'm to set an example for the rest of the group.''

B: ''Perhaps it seems that the boss does respond especially positively to me.''

C: ''I did get it there! What a bargain!''

Keep in mind when using the fogging technique that there is always room for more than one opinion. Rarely is anything so black and white that it worth arguing about. The goal of fogging is to stop the criticism. Later you can decide whether or not to do something about the situation that provoked the criticism.

TECHNIQUE #2—
ADMITTING THE TRUTH

The second technique of ADMITTING THE TRUTH is very effective when handling valid criticism.

The first thing we must do when handling with valid criticism is to accept it as valid, but not fall into exaggerated put-downs and negative self-talk. Avoid over-apologizing or over-compensating for your error.

ADMITTING THE TRUTH

WHAT IT IS:	A skill that allows you to accept your mistakes and faults without apologizing for them.
WHAT IT DOES:	Desensitizes you to criticism from yourself or others. Allows you to recognize mistakes as mistakes.
RESULT:	Once you accept your mistake, you can move forward, rather than becoming bogged down in depression and self-criticism. It also helps extinguish the criticism.
RESPONSES:	''You're right. I didn't complete the report on time and this is what I'm planning to do next month to ensure that the report is timely . . .''
	''You're right. I did not use the correct forumula in analyzing the numbers. Now that I know the correct procedure, I will rework the numbers.''
	''You're right. I probably didn't think it through carefully. Do you have any suggestions as to how I could improve?''

TECHNIQUE #3— REQUESTING SPECIFIC FEEDBACK

The last sample response leads us into the third and probably most powerful technique you can use in handling valid criticism—REQUESTING SPECIFIC FEEDBACK. With the use of questions, you can begin focusing on the future instead of dwelling on the past. It moves you directly into the ACTION stage and forces the negative critic to look at potential solutions instead of belaboring your failure. Also, it enlists the critic to be on your side.

REQUESTING SPECIFIC FEEDBACK

WHAT IT IS: Active prompting of criticism by listening to your critic and asking questions to elicit his/her feelings.

WHAT IT DOES: You gain information you can use, and you exhaust your critic's complaints. You uncover true feelings and discover common ground.

RESULT: You break the manipulative cycle of criticism by improving understanding and communication.

RESPONSES: ''What, specifically, did I do that...''

''If you were in my shoes, what would you do differently?''

''I'm not sure I'm clear about what your perception of the problem is. Could you please give me some examples...''

''Is that all you can think of right now that I could do to improve my performance?''

The basic skills of admitting the truth and requesting specific feedback help to extinguish the criticism and help you assess whether or not there is anything you can do about the situation. It also moves you directly into the ACTION stage, where you can take steps to correct the mistake or negotiate a compromise.

REQUESTING SPECIFIC FEEDBACK
(Continued)

Requesting specific feedback is also effective when confronted with vague criticism because in order to deal effectively with vague criticism, we first need our critic to clarify his/her criticism. By asking questions and requesting more feedback, we can reduce the criticism to manageable, behavioral terms. When coping with a vague critic, it is important to be genuine in your desire to receive information. It's helpful to use paraphrasing skills to help your critic clarify his/her expectations.

VAGUE CRITICISM:	ASSERTIVE RESPONSE:
"The report you turned in was really sloppy."	"What, specifically, did you find sloppy about the report?"
"You're not very much of a team player, are you?"	"What makes you think I'm not a team player?"

When asking questions of a vague critic, make sure that you use a neutral tone of voice and body language. It's not only the words you use but how you say them that makes all the difference in the world in how your questions will be received. Genuineness is essential. To get the point, read the two assertive responses above in a neutral tone and then in a sneering voice.

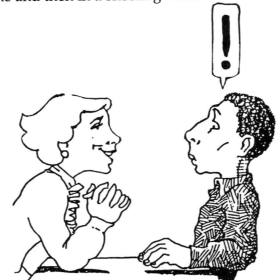

"YOU'RE NOT MUCH OF A TEAM PLAYER, ARE YOU?"

EXERCISE: HANDLING CRITICISM

A. Situational Case Studies

Here are several situations for you in which to practice your skills in handling criticism. Keep in mind the three stages of (1) Awareness, (2) Assessments and (3) Action and which technique is appropriate before you write out your responses.

1. Your manager wants to pull you off a project you have been working on for two months and give it to another person in your department. You think you have been doing a good job and want to complete the project. How will you approach your manager, and what will you say since s/he has not criticized your work directly?

   _____

   _____

   _____

2. A co-worker makes a derogatory comment about your work. What will be your response?

   _____

   _____

   _____

3. At your last performance appraisal, your boss told you that you could be doing a "better job." You want to ask her to be more specific, knowing that s/he does not like to be put on the spot. How will you do this?

   _____

   _____

   _____

4. Your best friend at work says that your attitude needs improvement when you feel you are doing the best job possible. How do you respond without appearing to be defensive?

   _____

   _____

   _____

5. Your spouse complains to you that you just don't help out around the house like you did when you were first married and that s/he is tired of doing the work. How will you address this issue and turn a potentially negative situation into a problem-solving opportunity?

   _____

   _____

   _____

EXERCISE: AUTHOR THOUGHTS ABOUT HANDLING CRITICISM (Continued)

Potential Responses to Situations 1-5:

1: ''I'm concerned that you are pulling me off of project x and giving it to Janet. Is there any particular reason for the change?'' (Requesting specific feedback)

2: Ignore the comment OR say ''What did you mean when you said...?'' (Watch your tone of voice: Be sincere). (Fogging or Requesting specific feedback)

3: ''I appreciated your feedback at my performance appraisal meeting last week. After spending some time with the evaluation, I noticed you wrote that I could be doing a ''better job'' in project management. Could you give me some specific suggestions on how I might be able to improve in that area?'' (Requesting specific feedback)

4: ''I'm not sure I understand what you mean. What have I been doing, specifically, that causes you to think my attitude needs improvement?'' OR ''What are some ways you can think of to improve my attitude?'' (Requesting specific feedback)

5: ''Perhaps I haven't helped out around the house as much as I could (Admitting the truth). What, specifically, would you like for me to do differently?'' (Request specific feedback.)

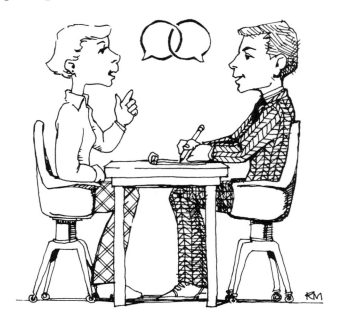

EXERCISE: HANDLING CRITICISM (Continued)

B. Personal Assessment of Criticism

1. Make a list of past criticisms of yourself that you assess to be unrealistic or unjustified and your responses to them:

CRITICISMS	RESPONSES

2. Make a list of realistic or valid criticisms of yourself and how you have or would respond to those criticisms:

CRITICISMS	RESPONSES

3. Optional Activity: Have a friend alternate giving you the unrealistic and valid criticisms outlined in #1 and #2 above and see how well you can respond to those criticisms. Your friend may also want to throw in his/her own examples to test your ability in assessing and taking action on unanticipated criticism.

EXERCISE: HANDLING CRITICISM (Continued)

C. Feedback on Your Ability to Handle Criticism

After responding to the Situational Case Studies or Personal Assessment Exercises, have a friend provide you with feedback in the following areas:

VERBAL	Excellent	Average	Needs Improvement
1. Did you face the real issue?	☐	☐	☐
2. Did you really understand the critic's feedback?	☐	☐	☐
3. Did you become overly apologetic or rationalize your behavior?	☐	☐	☐
4. Did you counterattack the critic?	☐	☐	☐
5. Did you communicate what you wanted to communicate?	☐	☐	☐
6. With the valid criticism, did you resolve the problem to the critic's satisfaction?	☐	☐	☐

NONVERBAL			
1. Eye contact	☐	☐	☐
2. Tone and volume of voice	☐	☐	☐
3. Facial expressions	☐	☐	☐
4. Body posture and gestures	☐	☐	☐
5. Nervous expressions (i.e. blushing, perspiration, etc.	☐	☐	☐
6. Other: _____	☐	☐	☐

COMMENTS: _____

_____

_____

MY PERSONAL ACTION PLAN:

I. These are my assessed strengths in handling criticism:

_____

_____

_____

II. The areas where I need to continue to improve my effectiveness in handling criticism are:

_____

_____

_____

III. Listed below are the situations and people from whom I can anticipate criticism in the future:

Situations: People:

_____

_____

_____

IV. Following is a list of positive self-talk statements I will utilize to counteract any negative thoughts I might have in coping with the situation and people identified above:

_____

_____

_____

V. Here are some potential statements I can use to deflect the criticism outlined in (III).

Situation: Response:

_____

_____

_____

A FINAL THOUGHT

A final thought on receiving criticism was expressed by Theodore Roosevelt who said:

> "It is not the critic who counts. The credit actually belongs to the man in the arena, whose face is marred by dust and sweat and blood—who at best knows in the end the triumph of high achievement, and who at worst, if he fails, at least fails while daring greatly, so that his place will never be with those cold and timid souls who know neither victory nor defeat."

To seek victory, is to risk defeat. It's a risk well worth taking.

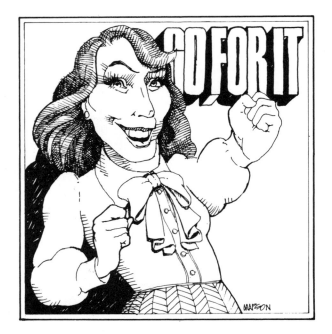

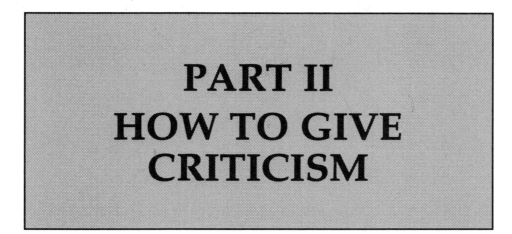

PART II
HOW TO GIVE CRITICISM

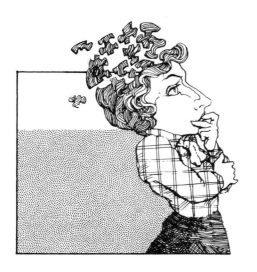

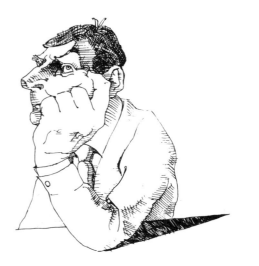

CHAPTER 7

BARRIERS TO GIVING CONSTRUCTIVE CRITICISM

Before we discuss the potential problems in offering criticism, let's examine your attitude towards criticizing others and some of the pitfalls you may encounter along the way.

Criticism Pitfalls

Check the attitudes that you carry into a situation where you need to criticize others:

☐   If I wait long enough, the situation will probably resolve itself so I don't have to get involved.

☐   Since I don't like to receive criticism, I can't imagine anyone else would. Therefore, I choose to ignore the problem.

☐   I criticize indirectly by using sarcasm or jokes.

☐   There never seems to be a "right" time to criticize, and I keep putting off giving criticism.

☐   It takes so much time to criticize effectively, I'd rather pick up the slack than take the time to correct another's behavior.

☐   I'm unsure of how the other person is going to respond to my criticism; therefore, I avoid giving it at all.

☐   I'm not perfect, so who am I to judge anyone else's behavior?

☐   If I give my boss negative feedback, it may be used against me at my next performance evaluation session.

☐   I let the situation go on for too long now, and I'm so angry that I'm sure I'm going to blow up and mishandle the situation.

The more of these attitudes you've checked, the more difficulty you will probably have in offering criticism.

THE SIMMONS/BRIGHT RESEARCH STUDY

The Simmons/Bright research study found that women found it more difficult than men to give criticism (30% versus 19%) and that people without supervisory responsibilities found it more difficult to criticize others than those with supervisory responsibilities.

Many people—51%—found it most difficult to criticize their boss. Regardless of who they were criticizing, people find that beginning the criticism was the most difficult aspect.

Factors Hindering Criticism

There are many factors that tend to prevent us from giving effective criticism. A basic barrier to offering criticism is that we may never have informed the other person of our expectations of them in the first place. This could be called the "mind reader's syndrome." Many times, we assume that others understand our expectations of them.

This is often the case with new employees. When hiring a new employee, many managers simply show him or her around the building and then to the new desk. They call this "orientation." However, the manager never really explained his or her expectations and goals to the employee. Often, a meager job description is permitted to substitute for a dialogue between the employee and manager.

The situation is worsened if a manager tells a new employee how happy he or she is that the employee has joined the company and that they were selected from a large pool of candidates. The underlying message to the employee is "You were selected as the best person for this job and should know everything about your new position automatically. If you have to ask questions, perhaps you're not as good as we thought."

When discussing how to give criticism, the first step we will feature is that we must set realistic goals and expectations with another person before we can fairly evaluate him or her (see Chapter 8).

Ignoring Situations

Ignoring problematic situations and hoping that if one waits long enough, the situation will disappear is the strategy adopted by many. Avoiding situations may be appropriate when the issue is trivial or when a problem is symptomatic of more pressing problems. However, ignoring situations is inappropriate most of the time, because most problems do not go away on their own.

Because of their intense need to be liked, some people refuse to criticize others for fear that they will not be liked. They tend to avoid conflict at all costs. They may also genuinely believe that they are not sufficiently competent to criticize others, because they are not above criticism themselves. But none of us is—so their excuse is a poor one.

Careful, well-thought-out criticism takes time. It may take less time and be easier to assume additional tasks rather than correct someone else's behavior. However, when we ''stuff'' our uncomfortable feelings or negative feedback, those feelings often surface later in upsetting ways.

> If people would dare to speak to one another unreservedly, there would be a good deal less sorrow in the world a hundred years hence.
>
> Samuel Butler

SHERYL: A CASE STUDY

Sheryl, an extremely passive woman, typically withholds her true feelings about problematic situations. She came home tired from work one evening to a kitchen table covered with a partially empty bread bag, an open peanut butter jar with a knife stuck in it, and an empty milk carton. She was angry with her son, the culprit, but he had already left with his friends. Her husband, Bob, walked in and, with ideal timing, asked, "What's for dinner?" Sheryl coldly replied that there was nothing left to eat, and they would have to go to the store.

She grudgingly dragged herself to the store and began taking her frustrations out on the groceries. Aisle after aisle, she slammed cans and boxes into the cart. Bob asked her what was wrong, but she snapped "nothing" and slammed more food into the grocery cart. Finally, Sheryl stopped in the frozen food section and lashed out, "I'm tired and angry that John left that mess. I don't want to shop, and I'm just plain frustrated and angry at the whole situation."

Bob started to laugh uproariously. Upon seeing her husband's spontaneous laughter, Sheryl also started to chuckle and asked Bob why he was laughing. He replied, "Do you realize that in the 20 years we've been married, you've never shared your feelings? I never knew if you were mad at me or what. I'm just relieved it's not me you're mad at."

A benefit of voicing criticism is that it can uncover problems early and can serve as the first step to solving them. In the long run, good criticism saves time. Without criticism, minor problems go unsolved and often grow into major crises. Criticism, if correctly handled, encourages both the critic and the party criticized to learn and grow.

Another potential barrier to giving criticism is the belief in the old adage, "no news is good news." Because we may be uncomfortable receiving feedback, we may project our feelings onto others. Consequently, we offer no feedback at all, either positive or negative. This is unfortunate, for most research conducted on motivation suggests that feedback is one of the biggest motivators for change.

CHAPTER 8

GUIDELINES FOR GIVING CRITICISM

First, in giving criticism, let's look at some positive results of criticism. Open criticism can relieve stress, permitting people to stop playing games of guessing at each other's expectations and evaluation of one another. Criticism can improve interpersonal relationships, for honesty promotes trust and paves the way to intimacy.

Criticism, correctly given, provides feedback that can improve job performance and promote continuing professional and personal development. Organizations that utilize criticism as a management tool enjoy higher levels of productivity and morale owing to their fostering a culture of openness. Openness is one of the components that can lead to excellence in organizations.

Step 1: Set Realistic Goals and Expectations

The first and most basic step we must take before we can give criticism is to let the other person know our expectations of him or her. If we have never shared our expectations, we have no basis on which to base our evaluation or criticism. A question every critic must ask him or herself is, ''Did I set up realistic expectations on which to base my evaluation?''

Paul Timm, Ph.D., author of *Successful Self-Management* outlines the characteristics of good goals.*

1. Be specific
2. Be realistic
3. Be measurable
4. Include deadlines
5. Be value anchored
6. Be written

If you establish and agree to realistic goals with another person, then you will find that when you do criticize that person, he or she will be more likely to respond to the criticism and act upon it. It is also less likely that the person criticized will take the criticism personally. Both parties must be committed to cooperation and a positive outcome.

> Not to alter one's faults is to be faulty indeed.
>
> Confucius

* *Successful Self-Management,* Paul Timm, Ph.D. — 1989Crisp Publications, Menlo Park, CA.

GUIDELINES FOR GIVING CRITICISM (Continued)

Step 2: Be Immediate

Once you have mutually agreed upon expectations, you need to observe the other person's behavior and be prepared to give positive or negative feedback, depending on the outcome of his or her actions. If someone has done a good job, don't just keep quiet: praise that person for it! Criticism can be positive as well as negative, and helpings of the former can help us tolerate doses of the latter. Give the feedback as close to the actual event as possible. Be short and specific. Select a good time, but don't save up your comments until you have a 15 minute litany to discharge. When giving criticism, you should not ask for a complete character change. It is far more effective to address one trait or issue at a time.

It is a good idea to be sensitive to timing when you are going to criticize another person. If he or she is already under a great deal of stress, you may elect to wait until he or she would be able to listen to you and do something about the criticism. You may want to put yourself in the other person's shoes and ask yourself how you would feel receiving the criticism at that time. Giving criticism requires compassion, insight, and tact.

Do not expect changes overnight. You need to be realistic about your expectations. That's why it is so important to set up mutual goals and be as immediate as possible.

If we wait and wait to give criticism, hoping that someone will change on his or her own, we will probably be disappointed. When someone doesn't change, we tend to lash out at the person in frustration. Simply because the wish for it has been on our minds so long, it is unrealistic to expect immediate change. Be mindful of the ''mind reader's syndrome.''

> Great Spirit, grant that I may not criticize my neighbor until I have walked a mile in his moccasins.
>
> Indian prayer

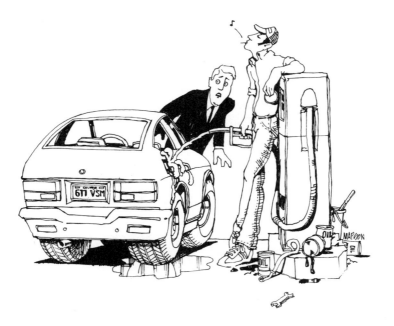

IF YOU DELAY CRITICIZING, IT COULD BE TOO LATE

GUIDELINES FOR GIVING CRITICISM (Continued)

Step 3: Be Specific

The Describe, Acknowledge, Specify, Reaffirm (DASR) script, or using "I" messages, is one of the best techniques in giving criticism. Normally, people have a tendency to use "you-blaming" statements, such as "*You* never turn in your monthly status report on time" or "Why are *you* always late to our staff meetings?" In contrast to "you-blaming" statements, *we* need to take responsibility to express *our* feelings and let the person we're criticizing know the *effect* of his/her behavior on us.

An effective formula for giving criticism is the DASR script. This is how it works:

Describe (the exact behavior you find bothersome)	"When you…"
Acknowledge (what you really feel about the other's behavior or situation)	"I feel…"
Specify (ask explicitly for a different, specified behavior)	"What I would prefer…"
Reaffirm (their worth or ability to correct their behavior)	"I have confidence that you can do the job correctly."

DASR Script Examples		
	Poor Version	*Better Version*
Describe	"You never get the data to me on time."	"When you turn in the staff absentee reports after noon on Monday…
Acknowledge	"You make me so angry I could scream."	I feel frustrated and rushed…
Specify	"Can't you get the numbers to me on time for once?"	What I would prefer is that you get the data to me by noon on Mondays so that Personnel can utilize the information for planning with the temporary agency.
Reaffirm		I appreciate your consistent attention to details and look forward to seeing your report next Monday by noon. Thanks."

If we had no faults, we should not take so much pleasure in noting those of others.

Francois La Rochefoucauld

What we often omit in this formula is the action-oriented specify step. A part of us really wants an apology or some kind of guilt-ridden response from the other person after we tell him or her how we feel. One of the most important steps in giving criticism is to specify a corrective action. This allows the person criticized to do something about the crticism rather than just defensivly reacting to our expression of negative feeling.

PATSY: A CASE STUDY

Here is a true example of how the DASR script was used in a personal situation. Ever since Patsy was in junior high, she and her mother had a history of conflicts, mostly small. As with many family spats, most of them were small misunderstandings. Yet, like a pebble in a shoe, even small things irritate over time. After many years of going back and forth on some minor issues, Patsy and her husband Joe decided it was time Patsy used her assertiveness skills with her greatest personal challenge—her mom.

Patsy sat down with Joe and her parents for about two hours to iron out their past differences. One of Patsy's compromises (compromises are a given when resolving most conflicts) was an agreement to phone her parents every other Sunday.

Several months after this agreement, Patsy called her parents on a Monday since she had attended a seminar over the weekend. Since her parents were both Christians and were brought up in the Church, they had reared Patsy with fairly strict views on Sunday observance, including no eating out, swimming, or other sports activities, and, especially, no work of any sort. However, this particular weekend was unusual in that Patsy made the decision to attend a seminar instead of her normal Sunday session of worship and celebration.

PATSY: A CASE STUDY (Continued)

When she called her parents on Monday, her husband happened to mention her seminar attendance and Patsy's mother angrily said, "*What?* You conducted business on Sunday? I can't believe you would do that." Dead silence. Patsy was stunned and angry. Who was her mother to judge whether or not she was wrong in attending the seminar? All of her training flew out the window, and she coldly replied, "Mother (instead of "mom," her more endearing term), I don't think you should judge whether or not I should attend the seminar without knowing the content." More dead silence. What was Patsy really saying to her mother? Even though it sounded fairly assertive, Patsy was really saying "none of your business." The conversation ended a minute later after perfunctory comments about the weather.

Patsy was devastated. She and her parents had worked so hard towards establishing a good relationship, and, in a matter of minutes, it appeared demolished. Once again, Patsy decided that she would put her assertiveness skills to work with the DASR script to deal with the situation. It took her three days to cool her anger and decide what she was really upset about. Then, she phoned her Mom to give her some constructive criticism. She wrote out notes with the basics of what she was going to say and had practiced her delivery and received feedback from husband Joe.

PATSY: A DASR APPROACH

Applying the DASR script, their conversation was as follows...

Patsy: ''Hi, Mom, this is Patsy.''

Mom: ''Hi, Patsy.''

Patsy: ''Mom, I just wanted to apologize for the way I reacted to you on Monday.'' (Pause) ''May I share with you how I felt about what happened?''

Now, Patsy's mom could have said, ''No need, I got your apology; that's all I wanted.'' However, by starting the conversation with an apology and implying that she was at fault, Patsy diminished her mother's need for defensiveness. Her mom replied, ''Of course.'' It's also important to note that Patsy did not apologize for attending the seminar, she merely apologized for her defensive reaction to her mother's statement.

> Patsy: (**Describe**) ''Mom, *when you* criticized me for attending the seminar over the weekend, (**Acknowledge**) *I felt* hurt that you didn't trust my judgment more. (**Specify**) In the future *what I would prefer* is that you ask me what the seminar was about and why I choose to attend it on a Sunday. This seminar really had an impact on me, Mom, and I hope that I can sit down with you sometime and share what I learned about myself and our relationship. (**Reaffirmation**) I love you and don't want something like this to come between us.''

Mom: ''I know Patsy, I cried for two hours after you hung up, but I could never have called you to apologize.''

> I can only know that much of myself that I have the courage to confide in you.
>
> John Powell

PATSY: CASE STUDY—AFTERWORD

Sometimes, it's hard to be adults with our parents because of our expectations of them. Yet, if we know the skills of how to give criticism in order to resolve conflict situations, it is a step and a risk we must take in order to deepen relationships. David Augsburger, in his book *Caring Enough to Confront*, makes this interesting statement, "Avoiding honest statements of real feelings is often considered kindness, thoughtfulness, or generosity. More often it is the most cruel thing I can do to others. It is a kind of benevolent lying."

It would be presumptuous to suggest that sharing honest feelings is easy and, of course, Patsy would have liked her mother to apologize, but the point of the matter is that the conflict was resolved and their relationship was deepened as a result. Patsy's willingness to share her true feelings *and* the specific behavior she would like from her mom in the future resolved the conflict.

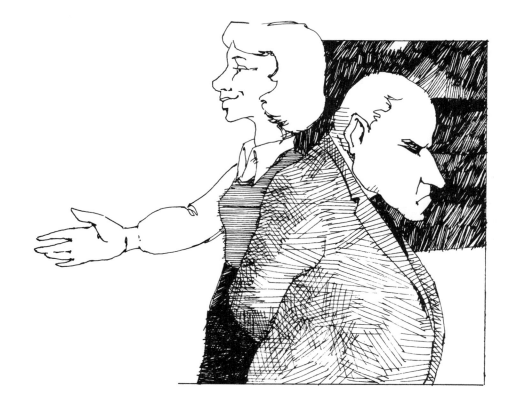

IT ISN'T EASY TO CONFRONT PARENTS

TWO WORK SITUATIONS

Let's look at two work situations and the various ways you could provide criticism. You identify which one is most effective and utilizes the DASR script.

Situation 1:

You are a sales manager in a non-commissioned retail store and have two clerks who talk more to each other than to the customers. You say to them:

> **Response A:** "Ladies, I'd appreciate it if you would pay a bit more attention to the customers."

> **Response B:** "Joan and Marcy, I'm concerned that your customers are feeling ignored because you are talking to each other rather than to them. I'd prefer that you talk with the customer during the sales transaction. I feel confident that talking with the customers will help to build the store's excellent reputation, and I'm confident that I'll be able to rely on the two of you to lead the way since you are two of my very best saleswomen."

> **Response C:** "Joan and Marcy, I'm going to have to write the two of you up if you continue to ignore the customers."

Let's look at each of the responses briefly. Response A began with an "I" statement but can be perceived as sarcastic. It also does not describe the unwanted behavior.

Response B is the best response, because it expresses the manager's concern and requests a specific new behavior. It also points out the rationale for requesting the new behavior and ends by reaffirming the two saleswomen's worth.

Response C is a "you" statement and is accusatory. The women will probably respond defensively and want to counterattack. Punishment is not a very good motivator in most situations.

TWO WORK SITUATIONS (Continued)

Situation 2:

You and your co-worker Michael work as technicians in the engineering lab. You provide him with the rough draft of the necessary technical changes, which he, in turn, enters into the computer system. A small problem has developed in that Michael consistently forgets to return your draft copy when giving you the final design print-out. You say to him...

Response A: "Michael, you can't expect me to remember all the changes I asked you to make. I need you to return the draft copy with the completed work."

Response B: "Michael, if you would do what you are supposed to do, I wouldn't have to bug you every 10 minutes for my draft copy. How many times do I have to remind you?"

Response C: "Michael, when you don't return my draft copy, I have to reproof. I'd appreciate it if you'd send it back to me with the completed work. This would save both of us time and enable us to implement these much needed changes more quickly in manufacturing."

Response A utilizes a "you" statement followed by an "I" statement. However, the co-worker has probably already lost Michael's attention, because the attack made him feel defensive.

Response B is definitely accusatory and sarcastic. It utilizes the overgeneralization "every", which automatically will flash a red flag for Michael.

Response C is the best "I" statement because it requests a specific behavior and provides a rationale for why the requested behavior is a "win-win" situation for all involved.

Rules for Assertive DASR Scripts*

	Do	Don't
DESCRIBE	Describe the other person's behavior objectively.	Describe your emotional reaction to it.
	Use concrete terms.	Use abstract, vague terms.
	Describe a specified time, place, and action.	Generalize for all time.
	Describe the action, not the "motive."	Guess motives or goals.
ACKNOWLEDGE	Acknowledge your feelings.	Deny your feelings.
	Express them calmly.	Unleash emotional outbursts.
	State feelings positively as related to goal.	State feelings negatively, making put-down or attack.
	Direct yourself to the specific, problem behavior.	Attack the entire character of the person.
SPECIFY	Ask for change in behavior.	Merely imply you'd like a change.
	Request a small change.	Ask for too large or too many changes.
	Specify the concrete actions you want stopped or performed.	Ask for changes in traits or qualities.
	Specify (if appropriate) what behavior you are willing to change to make the agreement.	Consider that only the other must change.
REAFFIRM	Reaffirm the other's ability to make the change.	Tell them your doubts as to their ability to change.
	End on a positive note.	Send them away concentrating on how you handled the criticism versus what they did wrong.

*Bower/Bower, *Asserting Yourself,* © 1976, Addison-Wesley Publishing Co., Inc., Reading, MA. Table 1, page 100. Reprinted with permission of the publisher.

EXERCISE: PRACTICE DASR SCRIPT

Change the following you-blaming statements into I-messages using the DASR script (''When you...I feel...what I would prefer...reaffirmation'').

1. Someone at work borrowed supplies you had purchased for a specific project. You-blaming statement: ''You always take things without asking permission. I don't know how much larger I need to put my name on those materials. Are you blind or what?''

   I-message _____

   _____

   _____

   _____

2. A supervisor from another department doesn't return your phone calls. You-blaming statement: ''I see now why you can never get anything done. You're too disorganized even to find my phone messages on your desk. No wonder everyone has to call you two to three times to get the information they need.''

   I-message _____

   _____

   _____

   _____

3. Your child does not clean up his/her bedroom as requested. You-blaming statement: ''Your bedroom is a disaster zone. Why don't you ever pick up your bedroom?''

   I-message _____

   _____

   _____

   _____

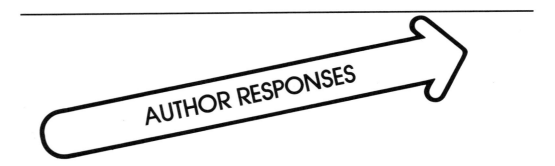

AUTHOR RESPONSES

AUTHOR RESPONSES:

Possible Answers:

1. "When you borrow my supplies without asking me first, I get upset because I purchase specific materials for the projects I have planned and when they are not here, I have to make last minute changes. What I would prefer is your asking me in advance about materials that you need and I would be happy to buy your supplies when I pick up mine."

2. "When you don't return my phone messages, I feel irritated because it delays me on the project I am completing. What I would prefer is if you or one of your staff members would simply give me a phone call and let me know when you can get back to me with the information I need. I'm sure this will help both of us be more effective."

3. "Honey, when you don't pick up your room when I ask you to, I really get annoyed. Let's work out a cleaning schedule that we can both live with, so that I don't need to bug you about it anymore."

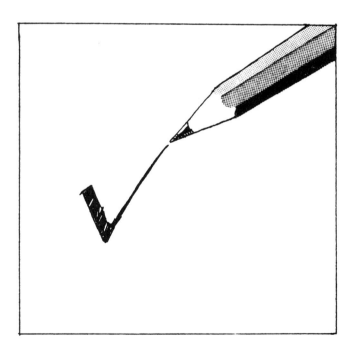

54

EXERCISE: INDIVIDUAL APPLICATION

- Think of someone you criticized in the past. What mistakes did you make? If you could handle it over again, what would you do differently?

_____

_____

- What interpersonal conflicts are you currently experiencing? What is getting in the way of your delivering criticism?

Person   Barrier

_____

_____

- Go back through the steps on how to give criticism and use the outline below to develop a plan of action to resolve your current situation. Implement your plan of action.

PLAN OF ACTION

1. *Describe* the situation and goals/expectations involved.

   Person _____

   Situational Experience/Goals _____

   _____

   What really happened _____

   _____

2. *Acknowledge* your negative feelings. List what feelings you have about the situation (see box below for list).

   _____

   _____

Vocabulary of Negative Feelings

afraid	devastated	hurt	offended
agitated	discredited	indignant	perturbed
annoyed	disgusted	inferior	put down
anxious	dismayed	insignificant	put off
apprehensive	distressed	intimidated	puzzled
ashamed	down	inadequate	neglected
belittled	embarrassed	irked	rejected
bewildered	enraged	irritated	resentful
bitter	exasperated	left out	seething
bothered	exploited	let down	troubled
burned up	furious	lonely	turned off
confused	helpless	mad	uptight
disappointed	hostile	outraged	unsure
discouraged	humiliated	overlooked	upset

3. *Practice.* Write out the criticism and practice saying the actual words you plan to use with a friend and get his/her feedback.

4. *Be immediate.* Don't save criticism up for a holiday. Once you have thought through a situation and the words you plan to use, pick a time and place to deliver the criticism.

When _____ Where _____

5. Be specific. *"I" Messages*—using the DASR script, outline possible words you can use.

Describe. "When you... _____

_____ "

Express. "I feel... _____

_____ "

Specify. "What I would prefer... _____

_____

_____ "

Reaffirm. " _____

_____ "

6. Implement your plan.

7. The result: *Improved relationships.* Remember, when giving criticism in personal relationships, there is never a single winner in an honest, intimate fight. Both either win more intimacy or lose it.

> To thine own self be true. Thou cannot then be false to any man.
>
> William Shakespeare

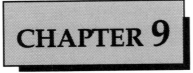

HANDLING RECURRING PROBLEMS

It is important to note that the DASR script is focused, short, and not conversational. Giving criticism in this manner is intended for first-time situations in which you are merely helping to put someone back on track about mutually set goals. Therefore, there is no need for two-way conversation. It is very similar to giving positive feedback; you merely give the feedback and move on.

However, there will be times when a situation recurs. Then, you will want to *discuss* it with the other person. Expect to feel some discomfort when having this conversation and be prepared with specific examples.

FIVE STEPS IN DISCUSSING RECURRING PROBLEMS

STEP 1: *Raise the Issue*

Identify the area of concern and avoid negative terms.

''I need your help with...''

''I am concerned about...''

STEP 2: *Describe the Specifics*

A. Avoid accusations and defensiveness by using ''I'' statements (the DASR script).

''When this happens...

the result is...

and I feel...''

B. Encourage the other person to discuss how he or she sees the situation by using open-ended questions.

''How do you see the situation...''

''Please share your thoughts with me...''

''Why is this happening?''

C. Summarize the other person's remarks to ensure that you understand his or her perception.

''So you see it as...''

''From your perspective it looks like...''

STEP 3: *Request a Change in Behavior*

    A. Mutually discuss ways of eliminating the problem.

       ''In the future, how can we...''

       ''How do you think this could have been avoided?''

    B. Actively seek the other person's ideas and suggestions. Encourage the other person to set targets for him/herself.

    C. Make suggestions, if you have any.

       ''Here's what I would suggest...''

STEP 4: *Agree on An Action Plan*

    A. Summarize what has been discussed and confirm your commitment. Show enthusiasm for the plans made. Be positive.

       ''OK, so I'll...and you'll...''

    B. Give the other person an opportunity to make any final suggestions.

       ''Anything else we should discuss?''

    C. Set a time and place for evaluation.

       ''When can I expect to see some changes?''

    D. Close the discussion on a friendly, upbeat note.

       ''I feel better now that we've discussed this, and I hope you do, too.''

STEP 5: *Follow Up*

    A. If the situation warrants it, you may want to keep a written record of the discussion and agreement.

    B. Evaluate how you handled the discussion and what you would do differently in the future.

    C. Set up a system for follow through (i.e. write the dates in your calendar, update your personnel files, etc.)

    D. Assist the other person in making the changes you have agreed upon.

FOLLOW UP

Follow up is a critical step in the process. For one thing, it makes clear to the recipient of the criticism the seriousness of the issue. Also, both parties can feel a sense of accomplishment when the agreement is kept and this increases self-confidence in both. Likewise, the recipient of the criticism is more likely to accept the consequences if he or she agrees to the Action Plan (step 4). By mutually agreeing to an Action Plan, there will be no reason for either party to be surprised when the issue is brought up again, either because the agreement was kept or broken.

Keep in mind that the only basic difference between giving criticism and coping with reocurring problems is a discussion. In chapter 8, we discussed how to give criticism to a person who has merely gotten off track. In that situation, you gently remind him or her of your mutual goals and expectations. In this chapter, we discused the situation in which you have already criticized the behavior as outlined in chapter 8 and sought outcomes which have not been achieved. It is at this point that you will want to have a discussion with that person about the reasons for the problem and agree upon an action plan as outlined in the preceding pages.

EXERCISE: PRACTICE CASE STUDIES

> The following case studies will give you a chance to try your hand at dealing with recurring problems.

| CASE STUDY #1: | **Performance Expectations Problem** |

A. Background Information

Jim Smith is a senior underwriter with 15 years tenure at Million Dollar Insurance Company (MDI). He feels that he is a good employee, and he has received good performance evaluations from his previous manager. Joanne Jenkins was hired from outside MDI to manage the underwriting department six months ago. She came to MDI with 12 years underwriting experience and has eight years experience managing underwriters. She brings to MDI both depth of experience and education. She is considered by most to be a "people person" and has high performance expectations of her employees. She has expanded the old MDI performance appraisal system and utilizes it to ensure top performance from those employees who report to her.

Jim Smith is a senior underwriter reporting to Joanne Jenkins. He is 58 years old and of his 15 years at MDI, 10 were spent in the underwriting department. Prior to MDI, he worked in a management position in a non-insurance related industry. He feels that he was unfairly overlooked and should have been hired instead of Joanne.

Jim is not sure why Joanne has expanded the performance evaluation form and feels that the old form was sufficient. All his past performance evaluations rated him as meeting performance standards. He is unaware of any current performance problems, although he has concerns about Joanne's high performance expectations. Jim dislikes criticism and can be defensive at times if criticism is not well-founded.

Two months ago, Joanne met with Jim to discuss and formally decide upon performance goals for his area of responsibility. Joanne sent a memo to Jim indicating she would like to meet with him on Friday to discuss his performance evaluation.

CASE STUDY #1 (Continued)

B. Joanne Jenkins's Role Sheet

You are the underwriting department manager. You have been with MDI for six months. You have eight years of experience as an underwriter and 12 years management experience. MDI is the first company where you have felt compelled to revise and expand the performance evaluation system. You are pleased with the new, expanded version and are seeing productivity in your department increase as a result of implementing performance goals and standards. However, you are particularly concerned with the performance of one of your employees, Jim Smith, who received ''rubber-stamped'' performance evaluations from his previous manager.

Since there was no substantive background on his performance, you met with Jim two months ago to outline his performance goals (you met individually with all the senior underwriters). You are dissatisfied with his work pace, although the work quality has been acceptable. You sense that Jim may resent you and the fact that he was not considered for your position. You are also concerned with his sensitivity to criticism. You observed his reaction to one of the department supervisor's criticism and do not want Jim to become defensive at your feedback. Your goal is to have Jim increase his work pace while maintaining his quality standards.

Jim is about to come to your office for the meeting you scheduled with him to discuss his performance evaluation.

JOANNE'S PLAN OF ACTION

STEP 1: *Raise the Issue*

''I am concerned about. . .
_____
_____

STEP 2: *Describe the Specifics*

''When this happens, the result is. . .
_____

and I feel. . .
_____

How do you see the situation?
_____
then, from your perspective. . .(paraphrase)''
_____

STEP 3: *Request a change in the behavior*

"In the future, how can we . . . _____

_____

"I might also suggest . . . _____

_____

_____

STEP 4: *Agree on an Action Plan*

"OK, so I'll . . . _____

and you'll . . . _____

_____

Anything else we should discuss? _____

_____

STEP 5: *Make plans to Follow Up*

"When can I expect to see some changes? _____

_____

_____

Potential Response to the Performance Expectations Problems:

"I am concerned about the performance goals we set two months ago. You have continued to provide excellent quality in your underwriting. However, you are producing 20% below the quantity standards we mutually agreed upon.

When this happens, the result is that our department becomes backlogged and overtime is accrued. Our department currently has 30% more overtime hours accrued than any other department at MDI.

I feel disappointed that you have not met the quantity goal we set together two months ago. At that time you agreed the standard was realistic.

How do you see the situation . . .

In the future, how can we continue to produce high quality risk selection as well as meet the goal of _____ number of applications processed per day?

OK, so I'll . . . and you'll . . .

CASE STUDY #2: Socializing

A. Background Information

Virginia Clark is a secretary in the marketing department. She reports to Jerry Drake, one of the regional marketing managers. Virginia has worked in the marketing department for 10 years and has reported to Jerry for several months. She is considered a good performer with good attendance. Everybody in the department likes Virginia, because she is social and interested in the well-being of other department members.

A typical day for Virginia consists of getting to work on time, going to the coffee machine and chatting with her friends and fellow employees for about a half hour. Virginia is a single mother and receives periodic personal phone calls throughout the day and makes phone calls in return.

Jerry Drake is an experienced manager with seven years of tenure at XYZ Corporation. He was recently promoted into the marketing area as a regional manager. When Jerry first came to the department he noticed a productivity problem due to the amount of socializing the employees engaged in on a daily basis. He met with the department one month ago to stress the importance of production and his concern with the amount of socializing taking place. Jerry noticed less socializing immediately following his comments but recently has seen the problem recurring.

A colleague of Jerry's, the manager from the accounting department, came to Jerry a week ago to state that she has repeatedly seen Virginia Clark in her department socializing. She is bringing this concern to Jerry because she thought he should know about the situation. She is also concerned about the precedent this may cause in the accounting department.

Jerry feels that it is time to confront Virginia about the situation and has decided to approach her on this problem.

B. Jerry Drake's Role Sheet

You are one of the regional marketing managers, a relatively new position for you. You have worked for XYZ for seven years, formerly in a small department. You are easy going, yet fair and consistent with your direct reports. You expect good performance and are concerned about the amount of socializing in your new department. One month ago, you held a meeting to discuss the importance of production and the effect socializing and personal phone calls has had on the department. Immediately following that meeting, productivity increased and the amount of socializing decreased.

However, several employees have continued to socialize after your department meeting. You are a bit embarrassed to learn from one of your colleagues in the accounting department that Virginia Clark has been bothering the employees in other departments. You feel the situation has gotten out of hand and is affecting the morale in your department and who knows how many others?

You know and like Virginia, who is very friendly and sociable. You feel it will be hard to confront her since she is newly divorced and is a single parent of two. In spite of this, you have a responsibility to confront Virginia about this issue, regardless of her personal situation, before it begins to affect the morale of your department.

You have decided you will talk to her about this problem and are getting ready to approach her.

JERRY'S PLAN OF ACTION

STEP 1: *Raise the Issue*

"I am concerned about. . . .

_____

_____

STEP 2: *Describe the Specifics*

"When this happens, the result is . . . _____

_____

and I feel . . . _____

_____

How do you see the situation?

then, from your perspective . . .(paraphrase)"

_____

CASE STUDY #2: (Continued)

STEP 3: *Request a change in the behavior*

"In the future, how can we . . . _____

_____

"I might also suggest . . . _____

_____

_____

STEP 4: *Agree on an Action Plan*

"OK, so I'll . . . _____

and you'll . . . _____

Anything else we should discuss? _____

_____

STEP 5: *Make plans to Follow Up*

"When can I expect to see some changes? _____

_____

_____

Potential Response to the Socializing Problem:

"I am concerned about the amount of socializing that occurs in our department. Although I am aware that other department members also socialize, I have specifically noticed that you are making 7-8 personal phone calls a day and that you are away from your desk at least 1½ hours a day. My concern was increased when a manager from a different department approached me yesterday about your visits to her department and her concern about how it may set a precedent in her department.

When you socialize, the result is that you may be affecting another department's ability to get their work completed as well as our own department's productivity by your absence.

I feel frustrated that the manager from the other department had to approach me, since I had made my expectations on this issue clear at the department meeting a month ago.

I understand that a certain amount of socializing is natural and even helpful in building team unity. You are very well liked here because of your friendly nature and I would not want to change your positive attitude. I would like to discuss your perspective and come up with a solution we can both live with.

How do you see the situation?

In the future, how can we prevent this from happening and set up mutual goals and expectations on socializing?"

PERSONAL PLAN

Now, let's apply the skills to a recurring problem you are currently experiencing. Complete the following personal action plan.

MY PERSONAL ACTION PLAN

I. Describe a recurring situation in which you need to provide criticism:

Situation: _____

_____

_____

People Involved: _____

_____

II. When and where would be the best time for you to provide feedback?

When: _____

Where: _____

III. What specific behavior(s) would you like changed?

_____

_____

_____

What are the results of the problematic behavior? _____

_____

_____

How do you feel about the situation? _____

_____

IV. What specific changes would you like to see as a result of providing this criticism?

_____

_____

_____

What are you willing to do to help affect positive behavior change?

_____

_____

_____

PERSONAL PLAN (Continued)

PERSONAL PLAN OF ACTION

STEP 1: *Raise the issue*

''I am concerned about... _____

_____

_____

STEP 2: *Describe the Specifics*

''When this happens, the result is... _____

_____

and I feel... _____

_____

How do you see the situation? _____

then, from your perspective...(paraphrase) _____

_____

STEP 3: *Request a change in the behavior*

''In the future, how can we... _____

_____

''I might also suggest... _____

_____

_____

STEP 4: *Agree on an Action Plan*

''OK, so I'll... _____

_____

and you'll... _____

_____

Anything else we should discuss? _____

_____

STEP 5: *Make plans to Follow Up*

''When can I expect to see some changes? _____

_____

CHAPTER 10

SOME FINAL THOUGHTS ON GIVING CRITICISM

Giving Criticism Via Letter or Memo

We have covered the basic skills in both receiving and giving criticism. However, there is one way to give criticism that has not yet been addressed—how to give criticism via letter. It should be recognized that it is far better to give criticism in person than by letter. There are several reasons why this is so: (1) you will not be able to discern how the other person is receiving the criticism, (2) you will have to wait for a reply, which can be stressful, (3) the choice of words becomes even more critical, because the recipient will have the opportunity to read and re-read your criticism. In verbal criticism, you only give the criticism once and then it is over.

Some people find that giving criticism in a letter or memo is easier because they will not experience immediate interpersonal conflict. The person criticized is unable to respond immediately and spontaneously. However as a result, the recipient will probably interpret the criticism as much more formal and final when received in writing. You will need to consider seriously if that is the impression you would like to leave. It may be appropriate to send a *follow-up* letter of criticism after you have discussed the problem in person; however, it is rarely best to *substitute* a letter for personal contact.

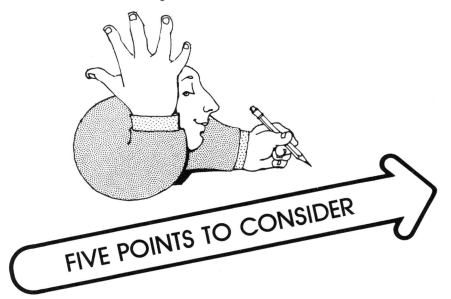

FIVE POINTS TO CONSIDER

FIVE POINTS TO CONSIDER WHEN SENDING A CRITICAL LETTER

If you do choose to send a letter, there are five points you will want to keep in mind:

1 Choose your words very carefully. You may want to have someone read through the letter before you send it. Make sure you are not speaking out of anger. Tone comes across even in letters.

2 Use a positive tone when stating why you want to solve the problem.

3 Include specific examples of the problematic behavior.

4 Suggest that the other person think over the situation and how it can be resolved. Invite the other person to call you if he or she has any questions. Indicate when you will be calling to follow up on the feedback so the two of you can resolve the problem.

5 Include positive statements in the conclusion of the letter about why you believe this will not continue to be a problem. Reaffirm the worth of the person criticized.

When Not to Give Criticism

Once you have decided on the form your criticism will take, keep in mind that there will be times when you will *not* want to give criticism:

• Do not give criticism when you are angry, stressed, or testy.

• Do not give criticism when the timing is bad or the person receiving the criticism cannot take action on it.

• Do not give criticism when you do not have specific facts or evidence to back up your feedback.

• Do not give criticism as a power play—to lower the esteem of the other or to make yourself appear self-important.

• Do not expect to see results from your criticism if you have not already established mutual goals or expectations.

SUMMARY

Giving and receiving criticism are difficult yet essential skills for each one of us to master. By opening ourselves to criticism, we can learn how to improve ourselves both personally and professionally. If we are completely satisfied with where we're at and are not willing to accept criticism, we probably will not proceed much further in our careers nor experience much growth and satisfaction in our lives. Thomas Edison once said, ''Show me a thoroughly satisfied man, and I will show you a failure.''

Providing others with honest feedback in the form of criticism can deepen our interpersonal relationships with them and can provide us—and them—with the tools necessary to improve productivity and self-esteem.

> There is a right time for everything...
>   a time to kill, a time to heal;
>   a time to destroy, a time to rebuild;
>   a time to cry, a time to laugh;
>   a time to tear, a time to repair;
>   a time to be quiet, a time to speak up.
>
> Ecclesiastes 3

The Serenity Prayer might serve as the last word on criticism:

God grant me the serenity to accept the things I cannot change;

the courage to change the things I can;

and the wisdom to know the difference.

NOTES

FOR OTHER FIFTY-MINUTE SELF-STUDY BOOKS
SEE THE BACK OF THIS BOOK.

We hope you enjoyed this book. If so, we have good news for you. This title is part of the best-selling *FIFTY-MINUTE*™ *Series* of books. All *Series* books are similar in size and identical in price. Several are supported with training videos (identified by the symbol ❶ next to the title).

FIFTY-MINUTE Books and Videos are available from your distributor. A free catalog is available upon request from Crisp Publications, Inc., 1200 Hamilton Court, Menlo Park, California 94025.

FIFTY-MINUTE Series Books & Videos organized by general subject area.

Management Training:

Human Resources & Wellness (continued):

Communications & Creativity:

Customer Service/Sales Training: